GRANDMA, WHERE DOES MY FOOD GO?

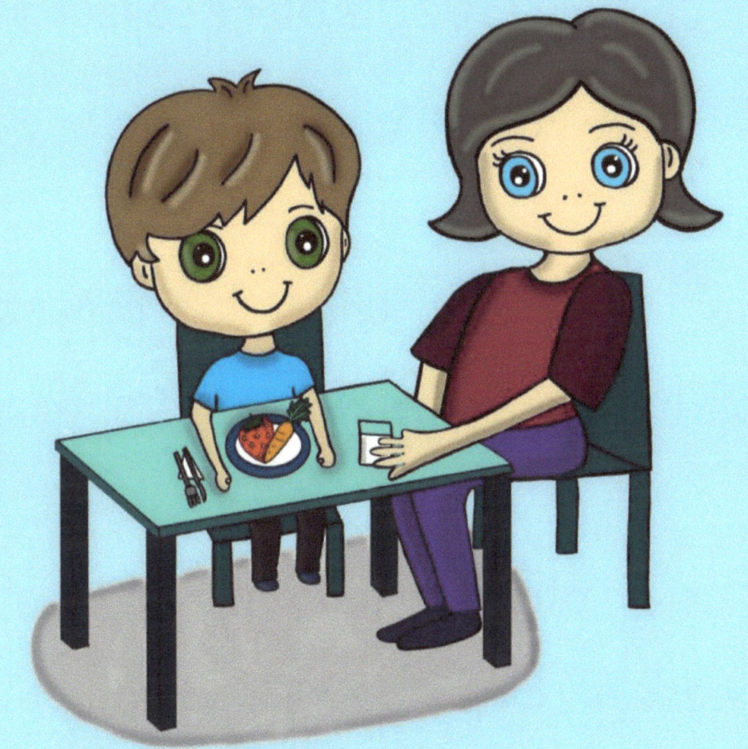

WRITTEN BY DIANE FAILOR ZAPACK

ILLUSTRATED BY CAMY DE MARIO

Many thanks to the beautiful women that have encouraged me to learn more about our digestive system.

I have to first say Thank You to my dear friend Lou who introduced me to Donna Gates, founder of Body Ecology and a dedicated pioneer of bringing gut health to the forefront.

Pam Craig, an amazing colon hydrotherapist, instructor and former IACT President (International Association for Colon Hydrotherapy) and Cathy Shea, my instructor. Her class inspired me to write this book.

Cathy teaches colon hydrotherapy internationally and is the founder of The International School For Colon Hydrotherapy.

I have so much love and gratitude for the knowledge shared with me.

Diane

This fun book is meant to be read to the smaller children by adults or older children, so they can start to learn the basic knowledge of the digestive system together.

Research says that approximately 80% of our immune system is in our gut also known as the digestive system.
A very important reason to understand and support a healthy lifestyle.

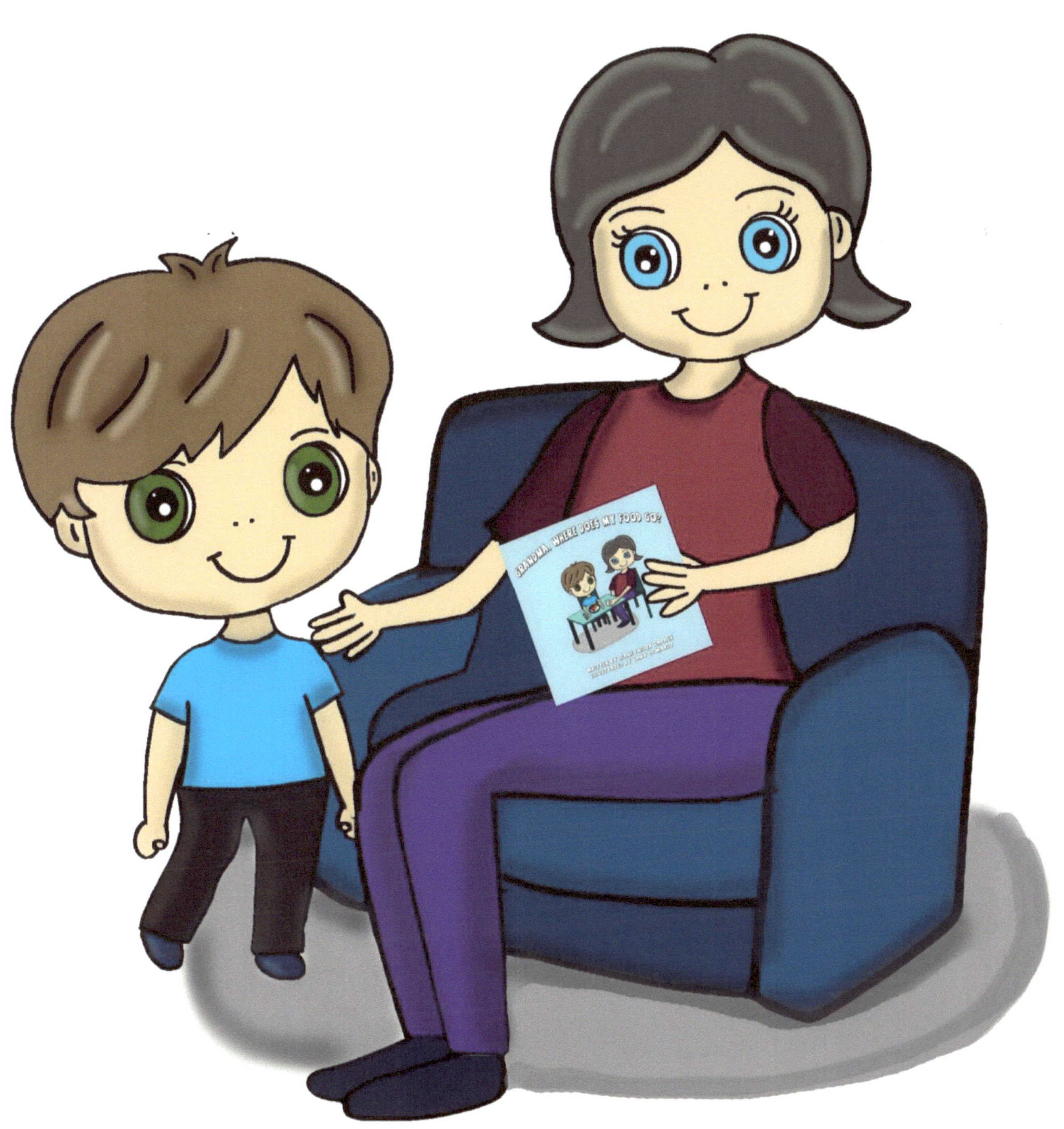

GRANDMA, WHERE DOES MY FOOD GO?

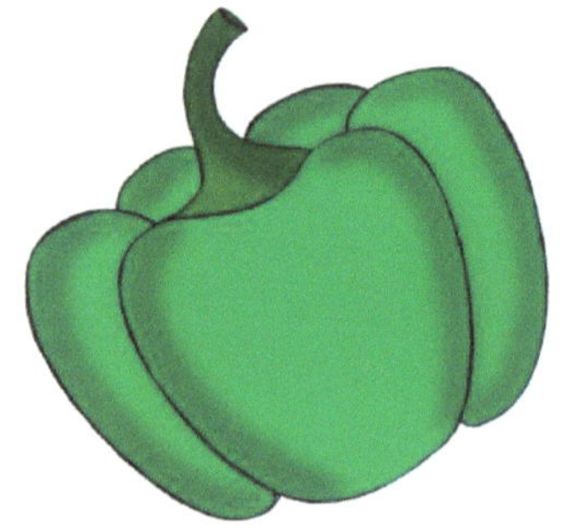

Once upon a time there was a very curious little boy who loved to eat.

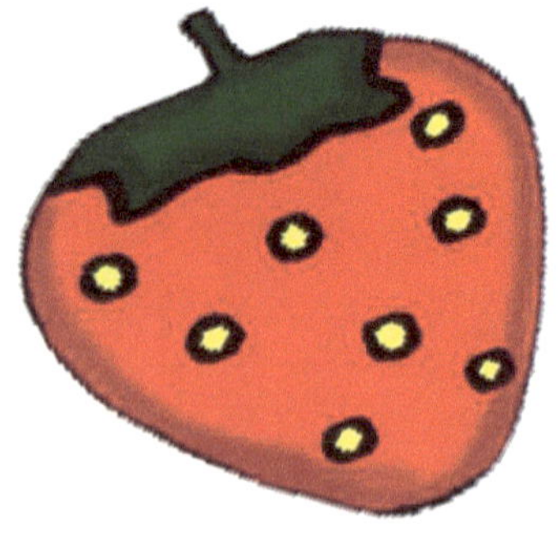

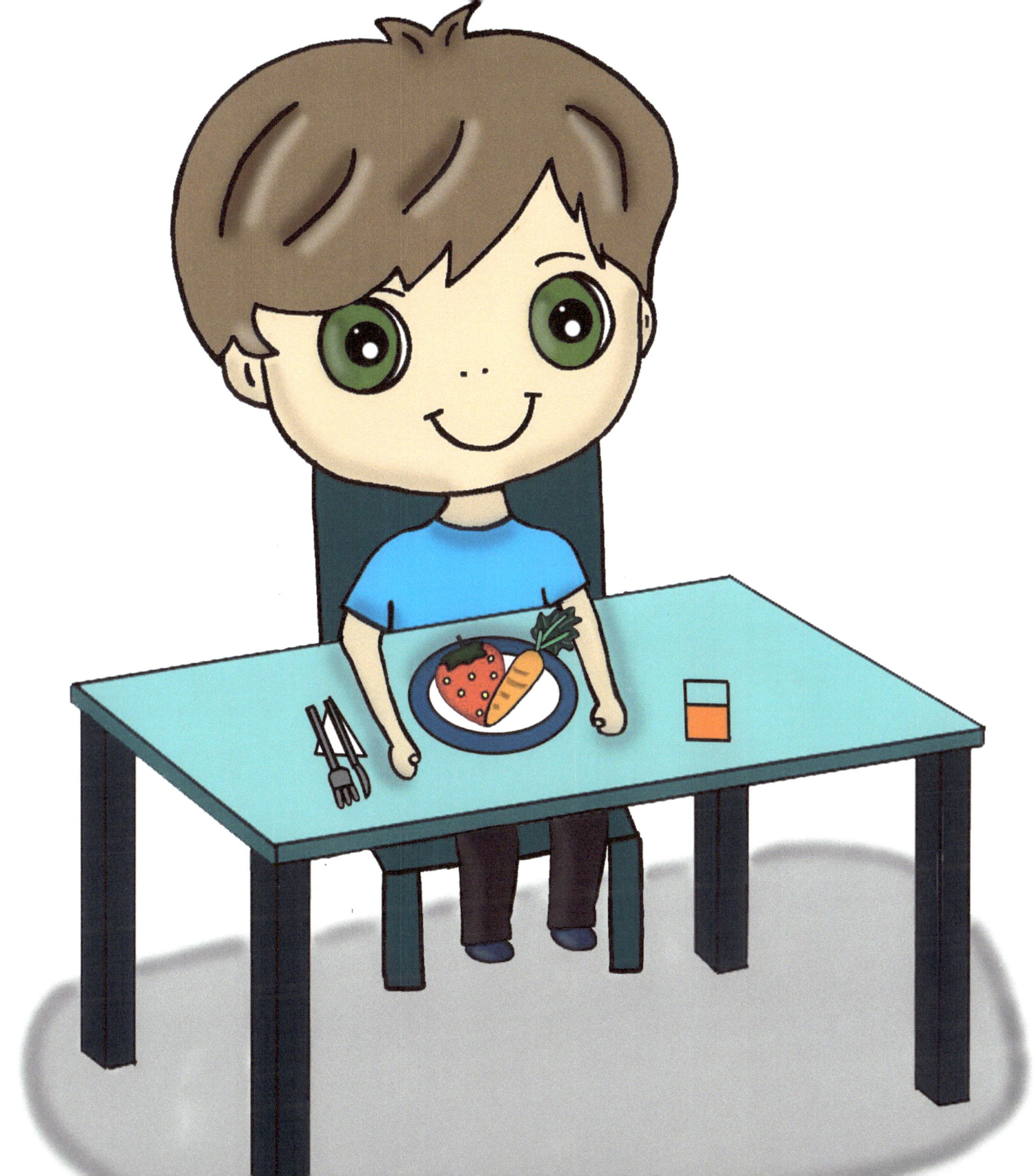

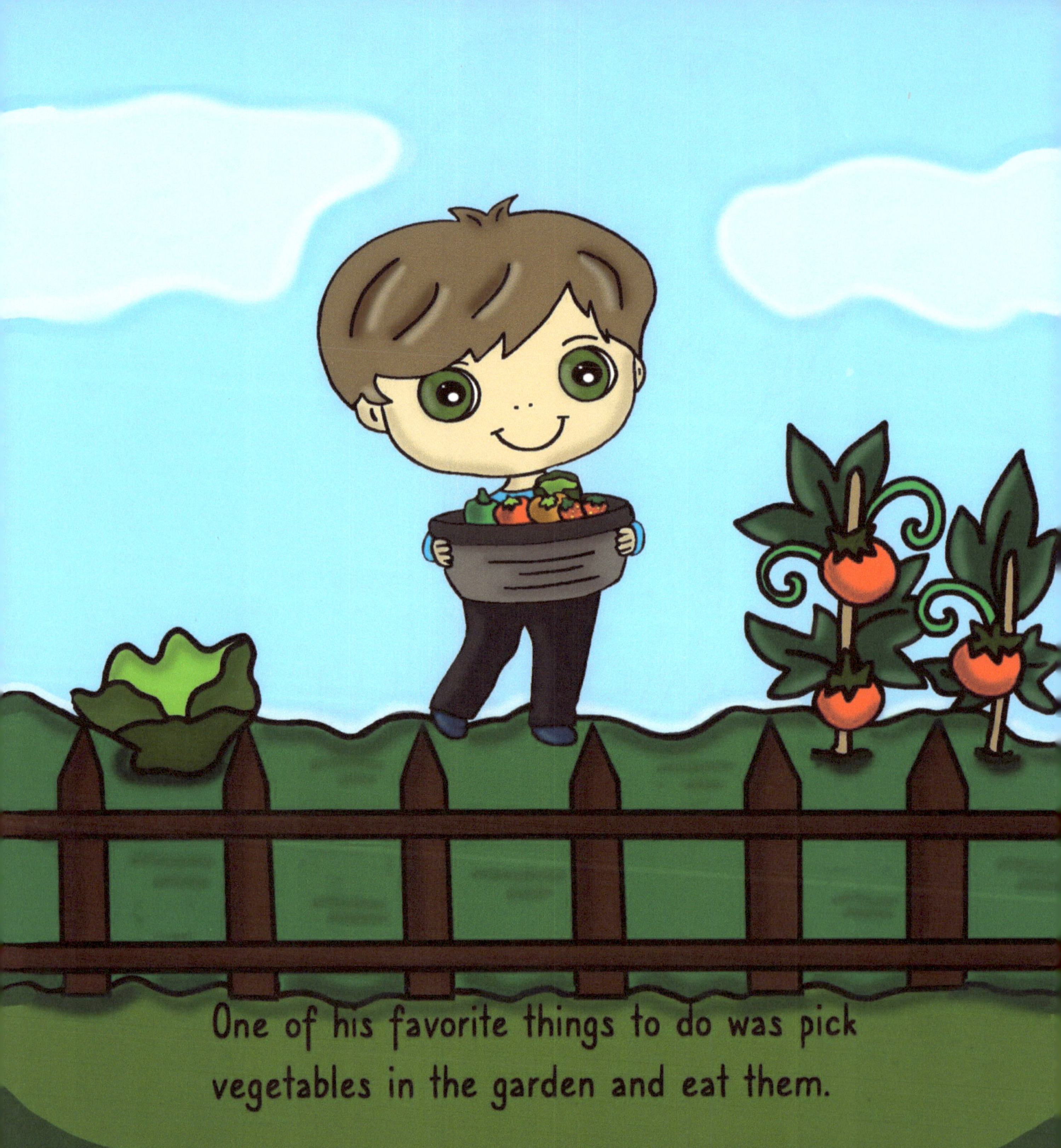
One of his favorite things to do was pick
vegetables in the garden and eat them.

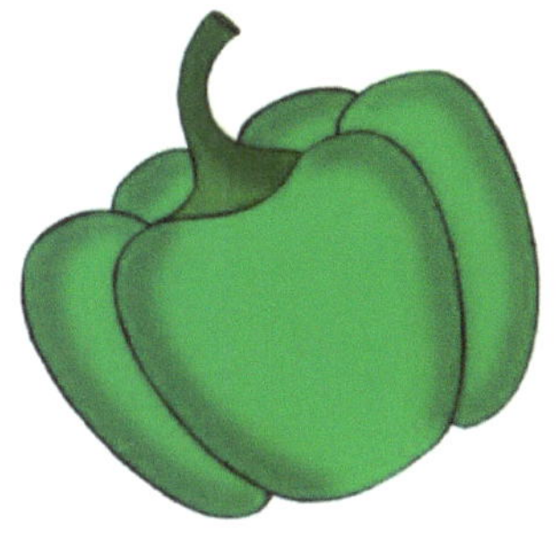 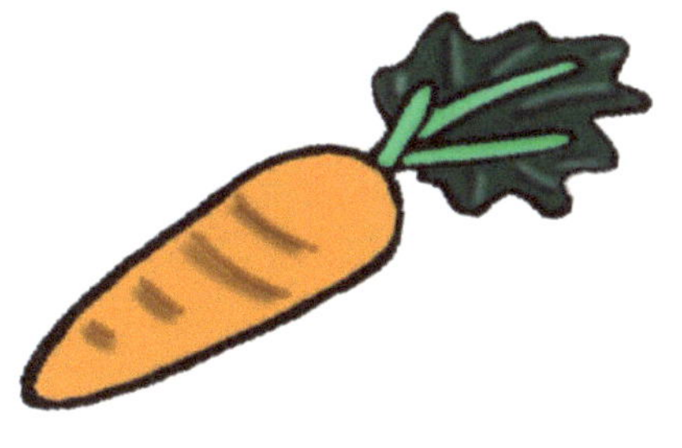

He tried so hard to figure out what happened
to his food after he swallowed it, but he couldn't
figure it out.

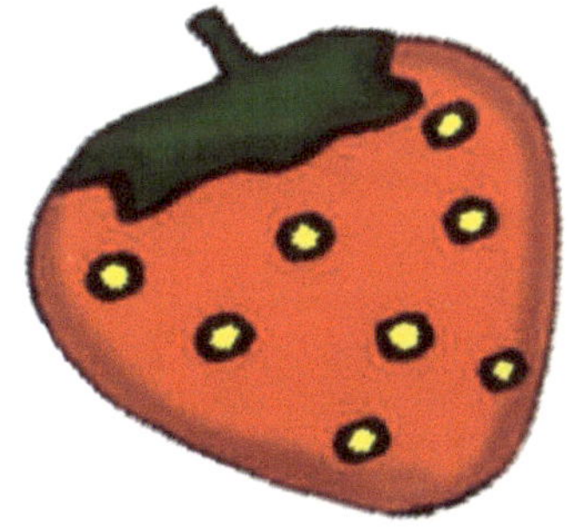

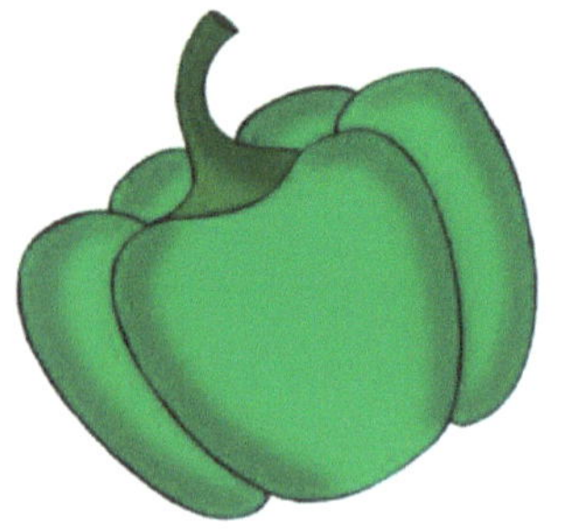

So he went to his favorite person in the whole
world to find the answer...His Grandma!

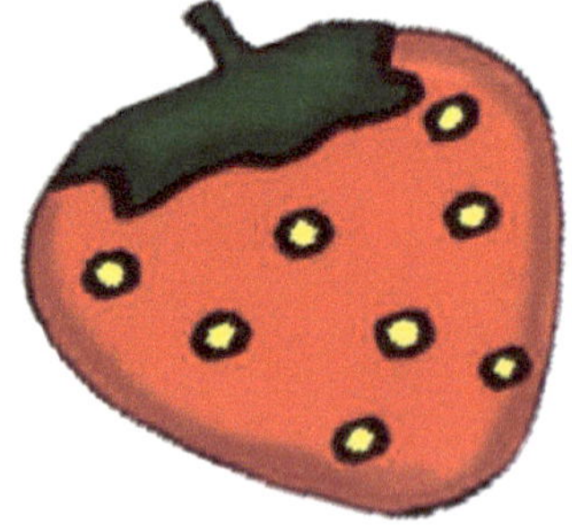

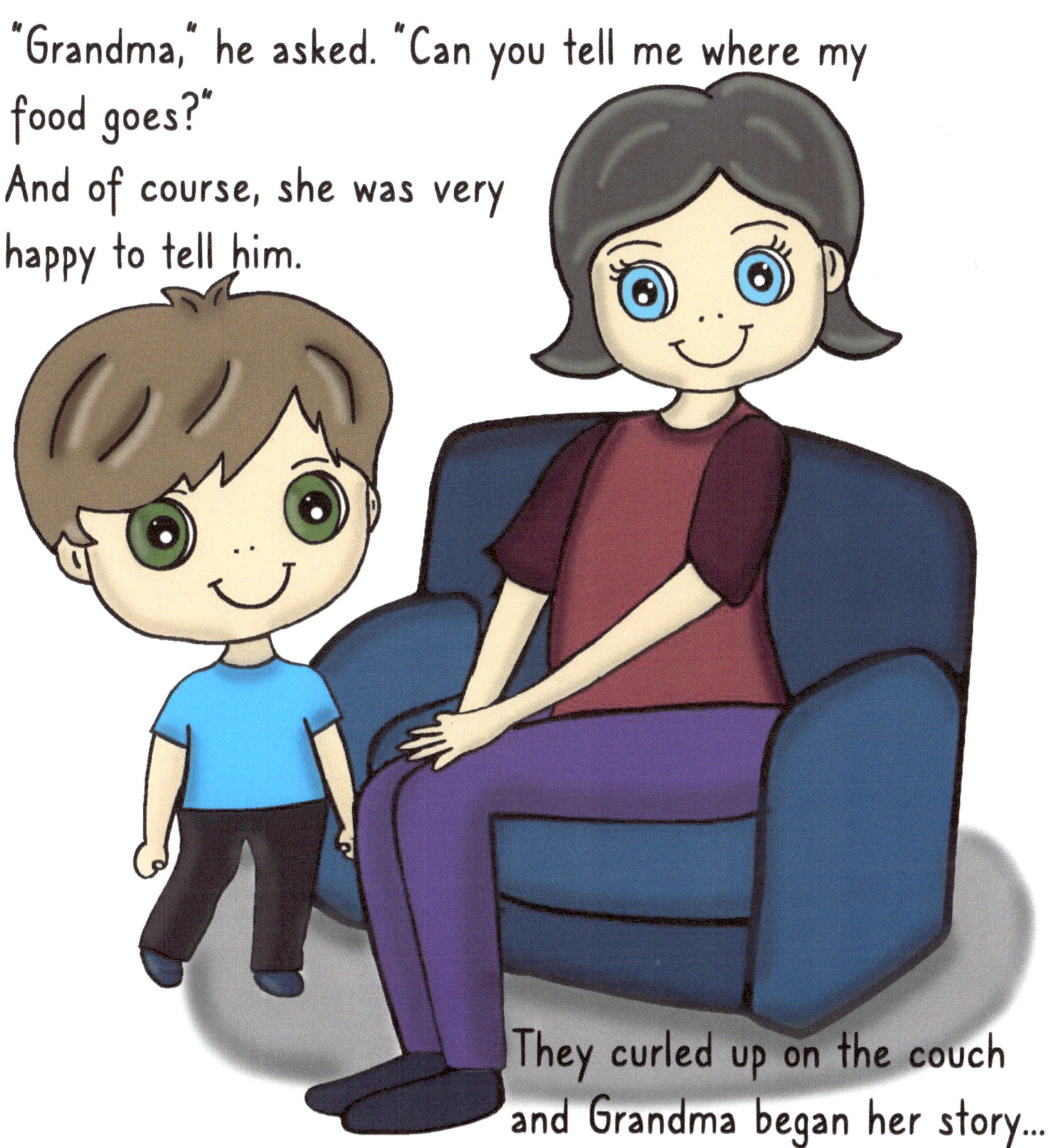
"Grandma," he asked. "Can you tell me where my food goes?"
And of course, she was very happy to tell him.
They curled up on the couch and Grandma began her story...

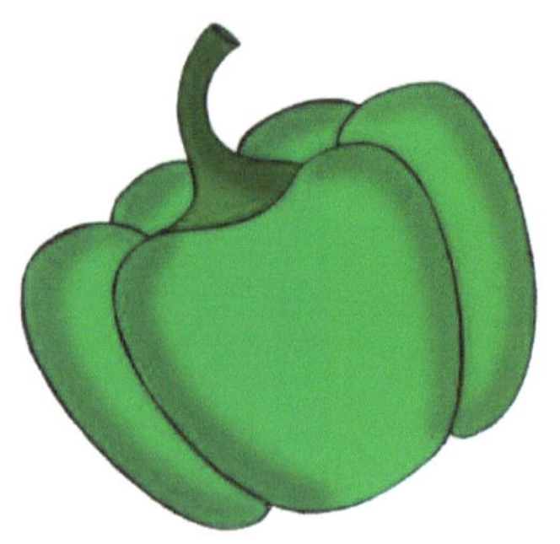

"Let's start at the beginning," said Grandma. "First we start with a rainbow of fresh vegetables, fruits, grains and proteins. Our eyes will tell our brain exactly what we are about to eat. Then the brain makes a list of everything so it can tell your body organs what they need to do.

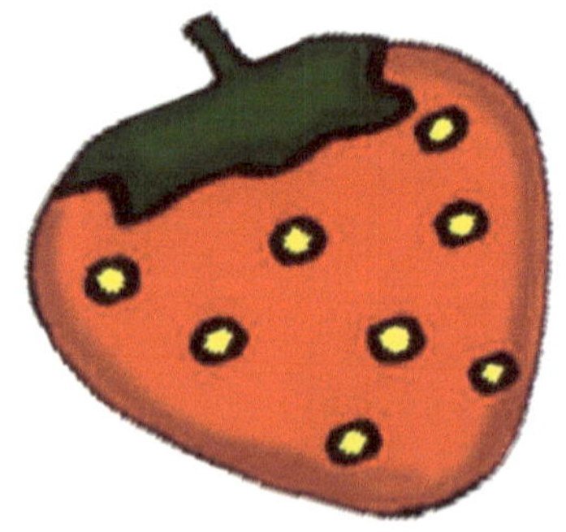

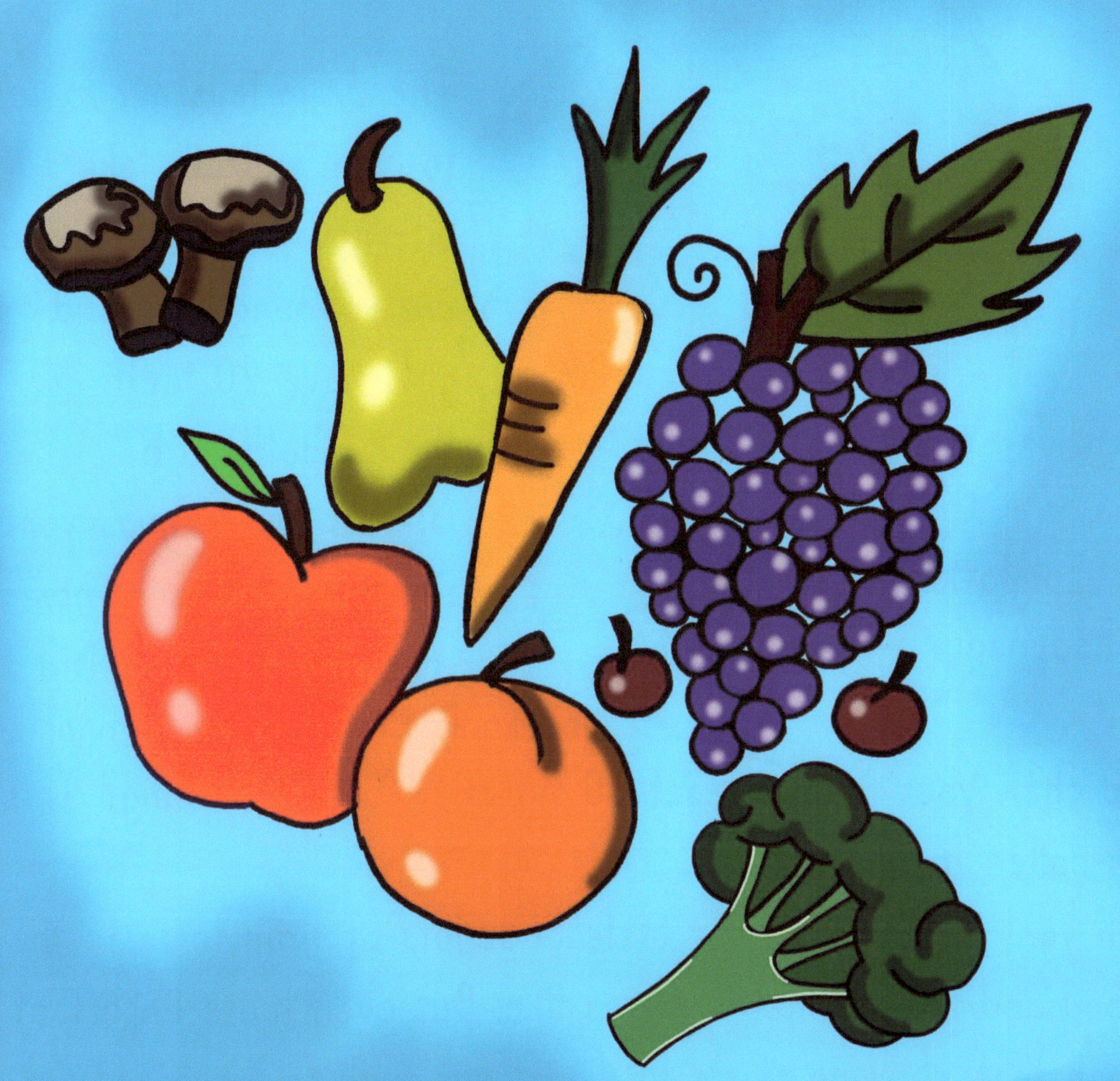

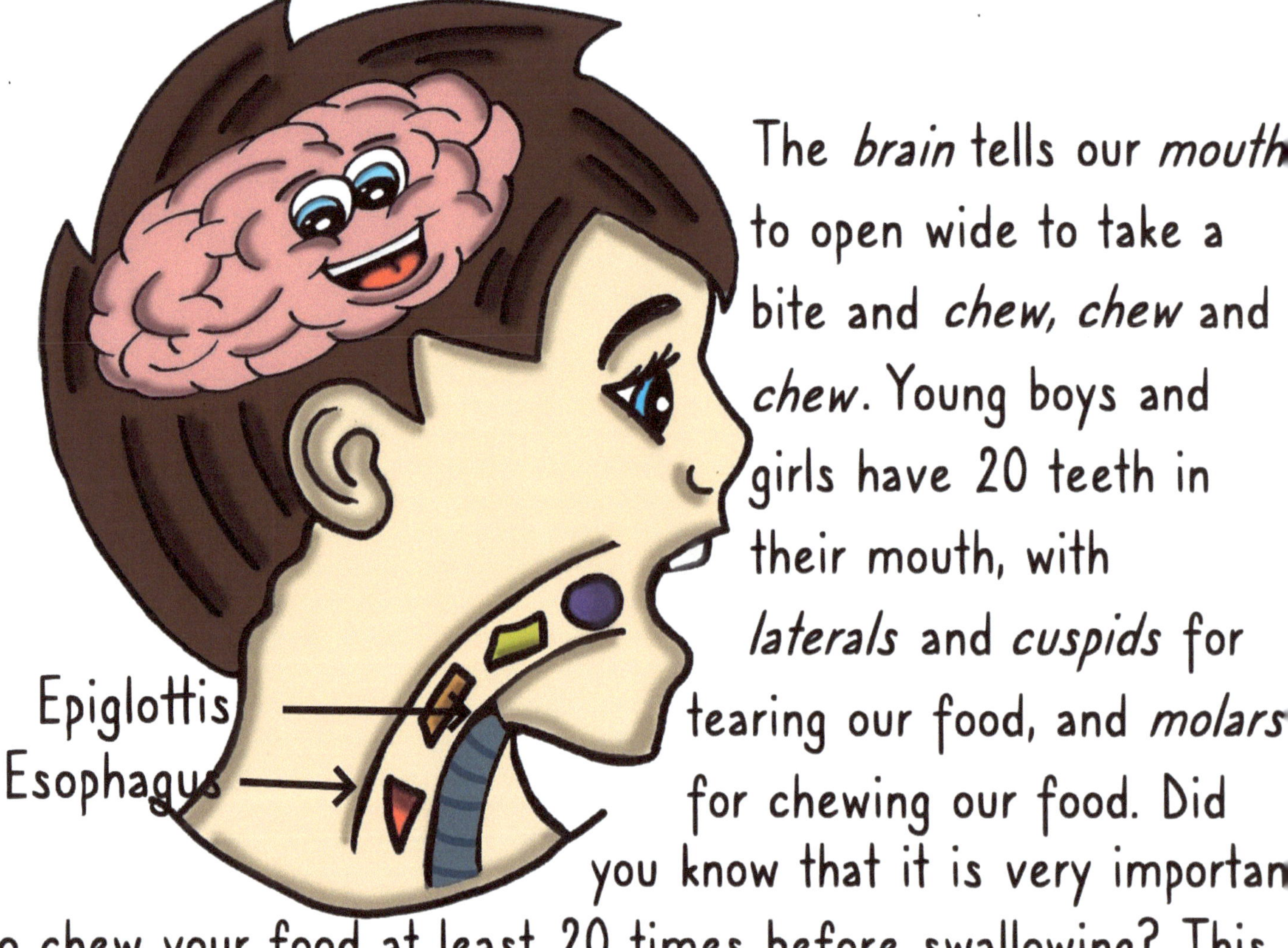

The *brain* tells our *mouth* to open wide to take a bite and *chew, chew* and *chew*. Young boys and girls have 20 teeth in their mouth, with *laterals* and *cuspids* for tearing our food, and *molars* for chewing our food. Did you know that it is very important to chew your food at least 20 times before swallowing? This is called *mastication.*

Oh yes! It also gives our taste buds lots of time to taste the food and tell us what it tastes like. But even more important than that, chewing starts to digest our food to prepare it for

its journey to our bellies, which is also called our *stomach*.
There are three special glands in our mouth named the
parotid, the *sublingual,* and the *submandibular.* These very
special glands release a fluid called *saliva.* This helps to
start digesting our food, or make it smaller. This will make
it easier for our *tongue* to move the food to the back of our
mouth to *swallow.* Next it passes a very, very important door
called the *epiglottis.* This door protects our food from going
down our windpipe so we don't choke.

Our friend *peristalsis* rhythmically squeezes the food towards
the stomach through the *esophagus.*

What a fun ride down the esophagus straight through the
lower esophageal sphincter doorway, and splashing right into
the stomach.

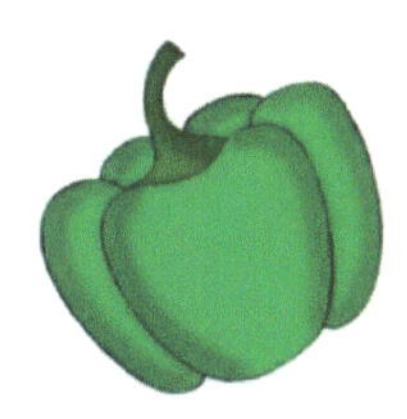 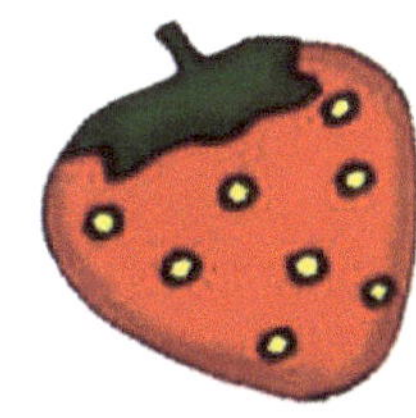 

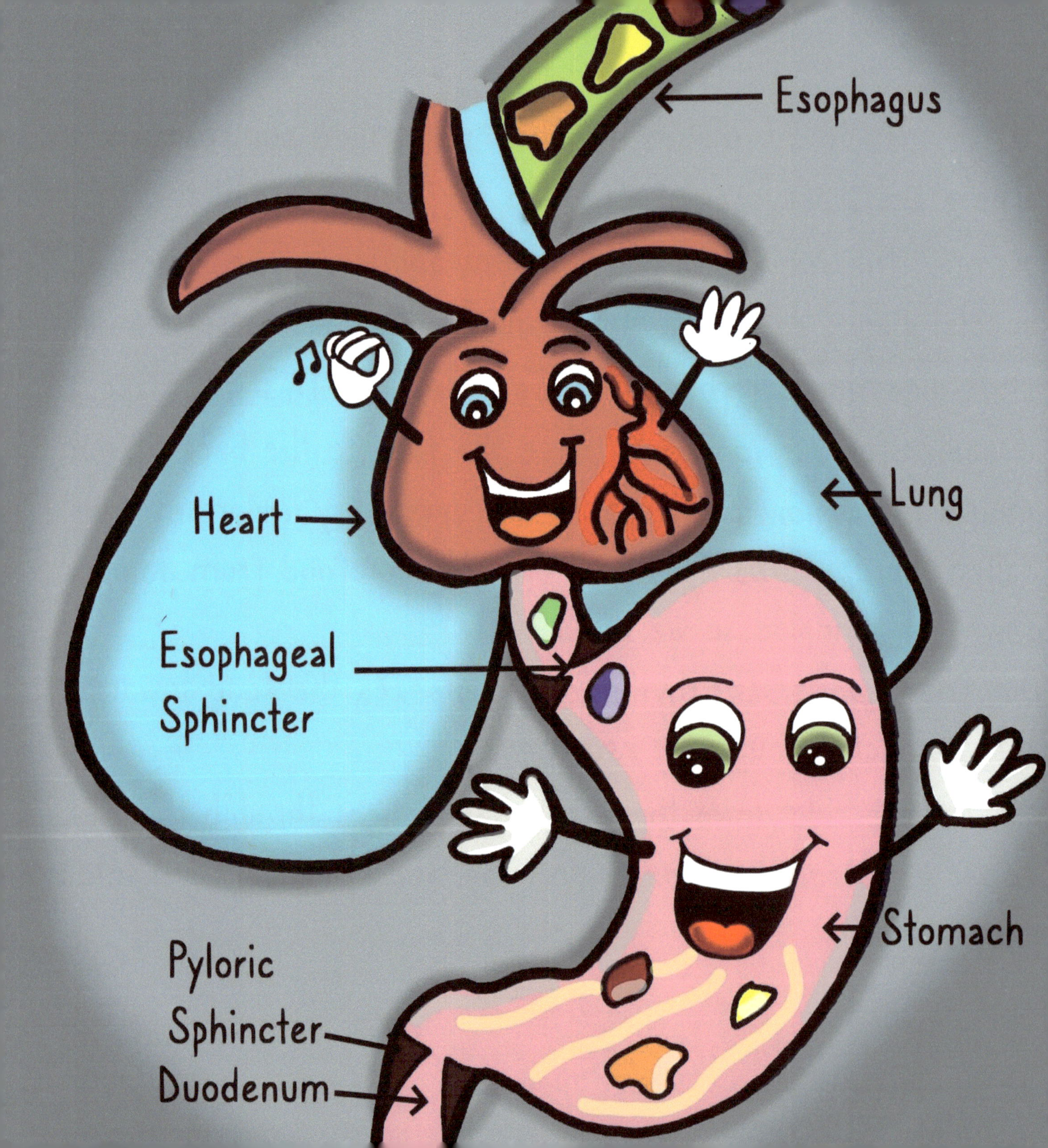

Esophagus
Lung
Heart
Esophageal
Sphincter
Stomach
Pyloric
Sphincter
Duodenum

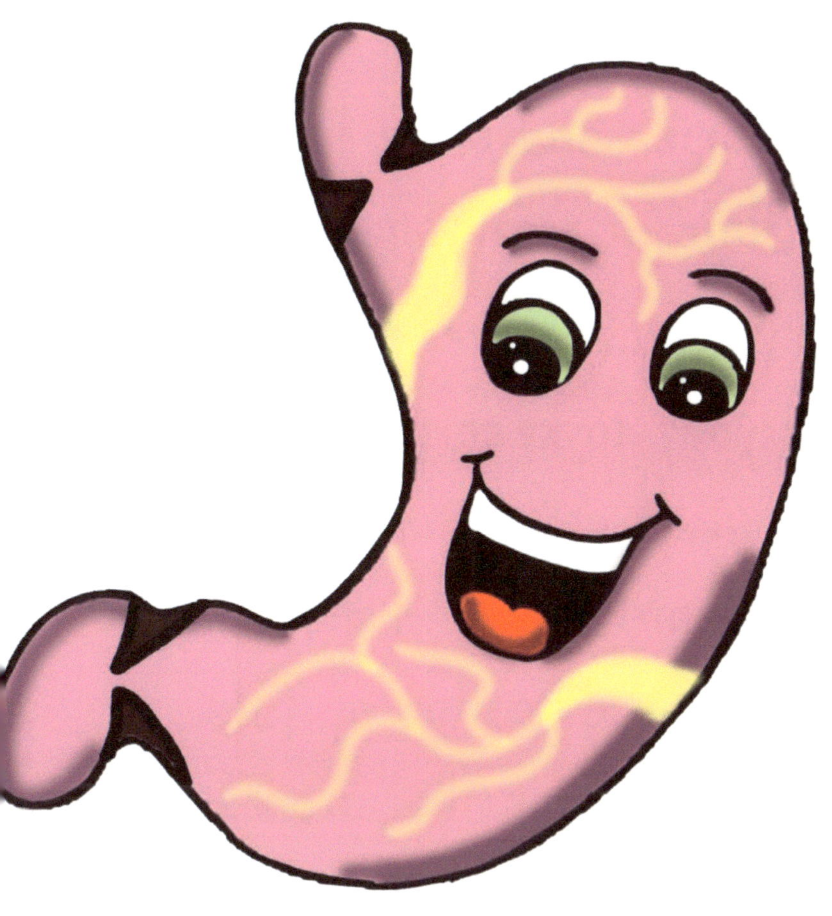

The *stomach* is full of gastric juices called *hydrochloric acid.* This acid is designed especially for breaking down our food so it can continue its exciting journey.

The long yellow lines that look like water slides are called *rugae.* They have the job of expanding our stomach when we eat a lot and bring it back to its normal size when it's empty. Our food is now much softer, almost liquid, and is called *chyme.* Now it is ready to leave the stomach and pass through the *pyloric sphincter* into the *duodenum.*

This is a doorway that will open and close to let a little *chyme* pass through at a time in small squirts.

There are three organs that became very dear friends. They help each other everyday to keep our body in balance. Their names are *liver*, *gallbladder*, and *pancreas*.

The *liver* is the biggest organ. Its role in digestion is secreting *bile* which aids in the digestion of fats.

The *gallbladder* is a very small organ that stores the *bile* from the *liver* and releases it as needed in to the *small intestine.*

The *pancreas* produces hormones such as insulin to balance our blood sugar and makes extra digestive enzymes if we need them.

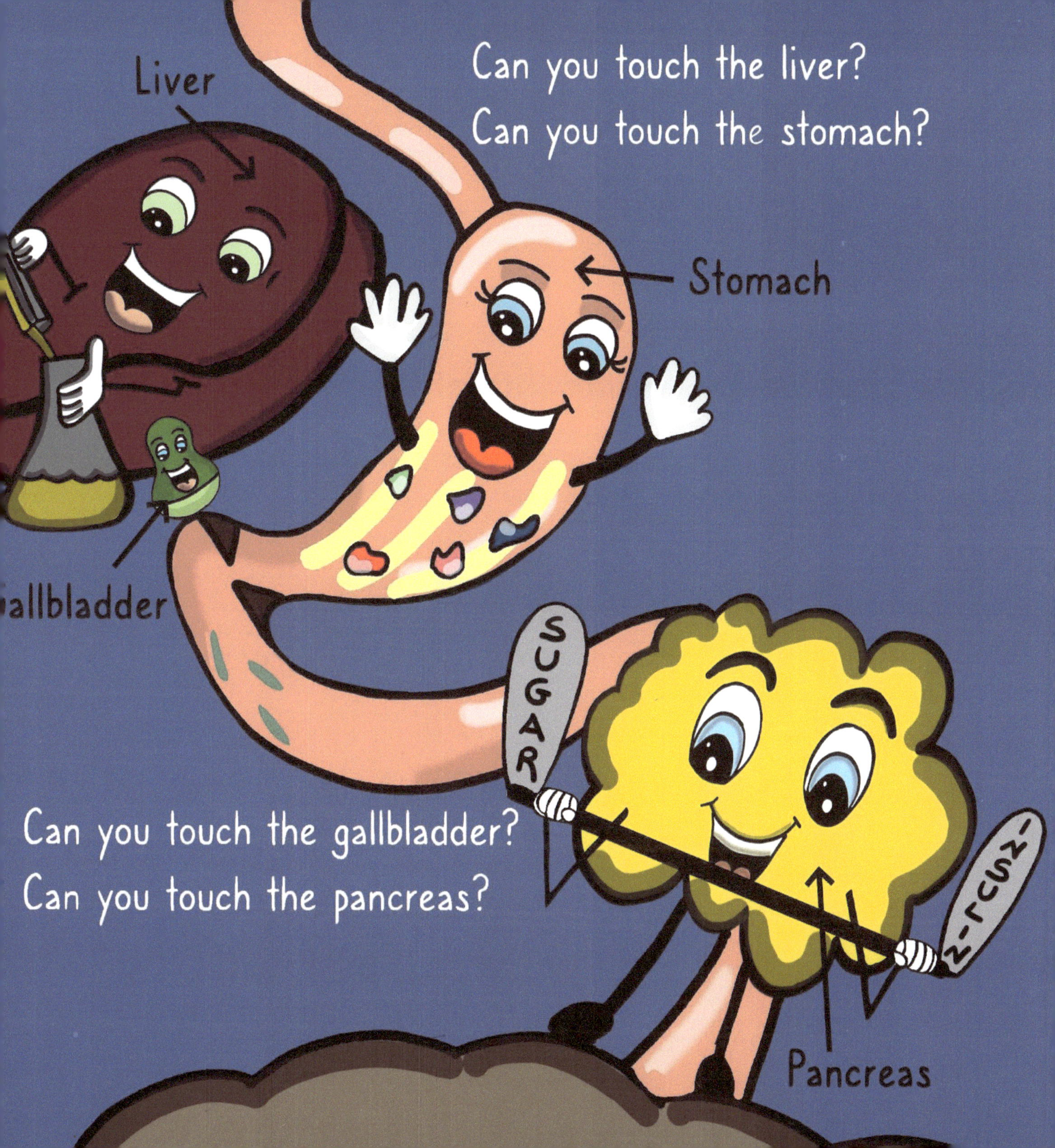

Can you touch the liver?
Can you touch the stomach?
Liver
Stomach
Gallbladder
Can you touch the gallbladder?
Can you touch the pancreas?
SUGAR
INSULIN
Pancreas

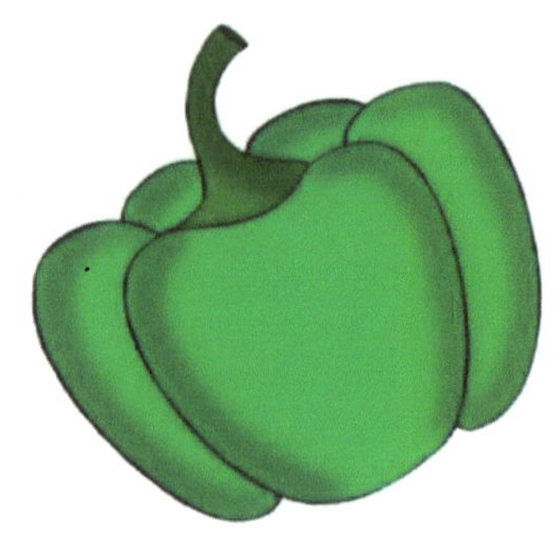

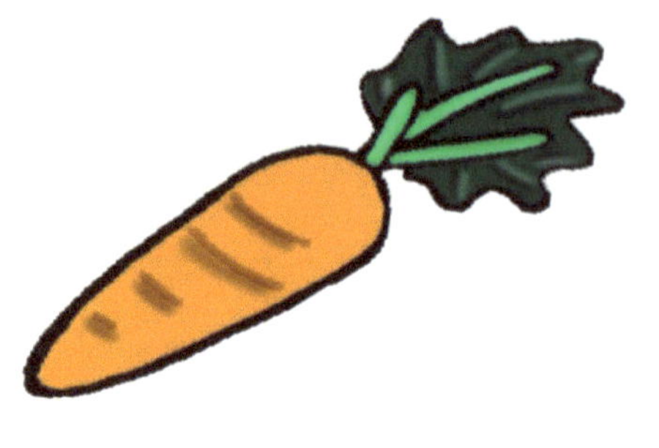

Now we have a wild ride through the *small intestine!* Starting with the *duodenum,* around the *jejunum* and finally through the *ileum.*

This is where the *digestion* continues and the *absorption* begins. Sending nutrients to your bloodstream and traveling to all the cells of the body through little fingers called *villi.* Under the fingers called *villi* we have a very big family of *immune cells* that need fresh food to keep us healthy.

Can you follow the *small intestine* through the maze all the way to the *ileocecal valve?*

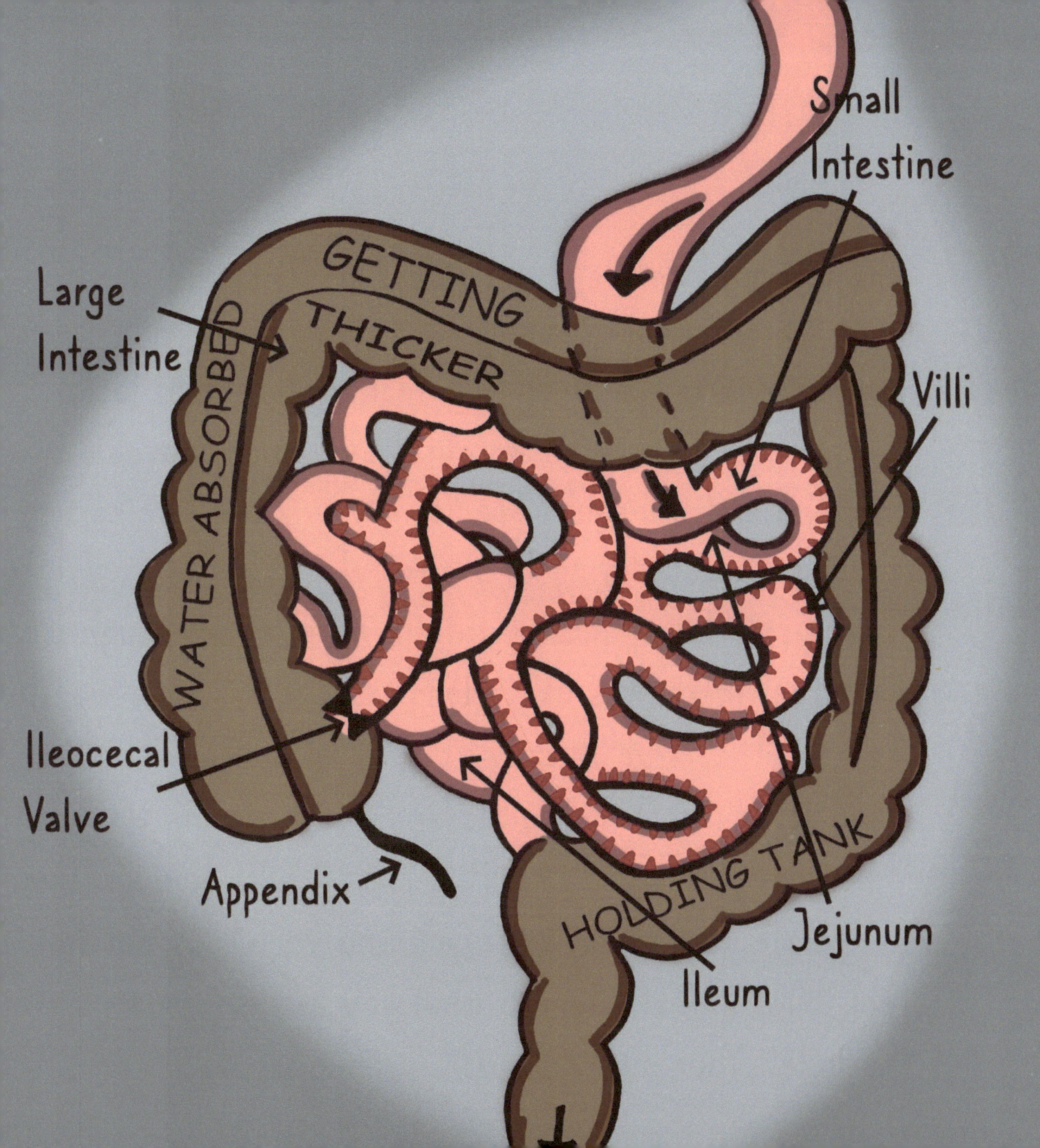

Small Intestine
Large Intestine
GETTING THICKER
WATER ABSORBED
Villi
Ileocecal Valve
Appendix
HOLDING TANK
Ileum
Jejunum

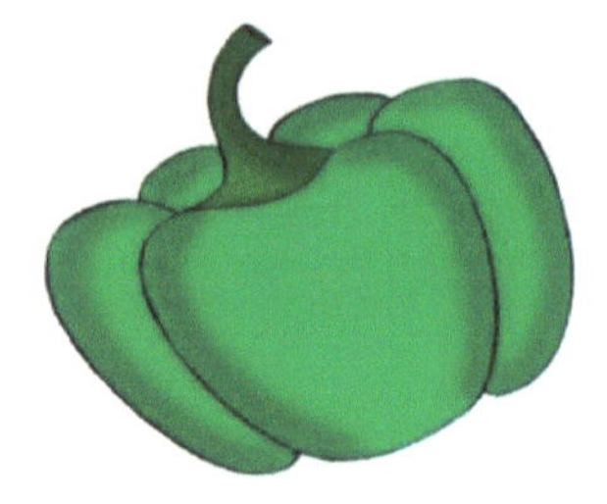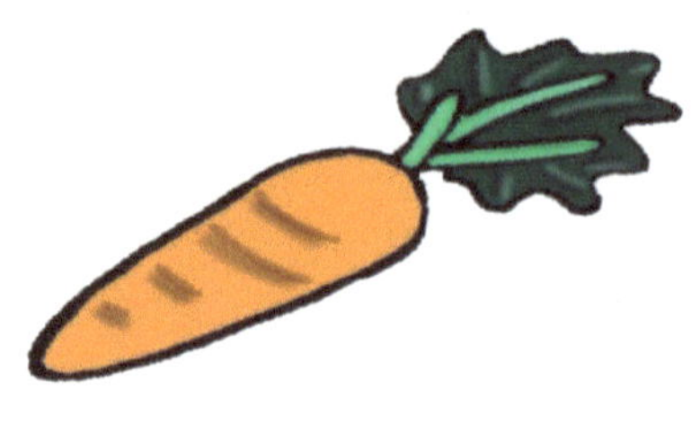

This brings us to the *large intestine...* There is so much going on here!

Your *appendix* is a small but mighty organ that looks like a worm. It keeps a watchful eye on the *large intestine* and will squirt special *lymph fluid* to clean up any bad bacteria trying to sneak by!

There are a lot of movements in here, even though we don't feel them! It's like a long train ride all the way to the end. The *large intestine* drinks up and absorbs the liquid from the food you ate and drank. Then, it sends it through your *veins* like little rivers, back to your liver to hydrate you, which helps you and your body not to feel thirsty. What's left is what you see in the toilet... Your *poop (fecal)!*

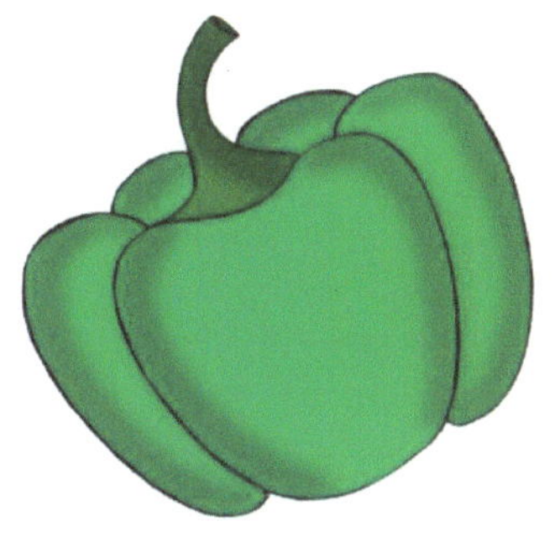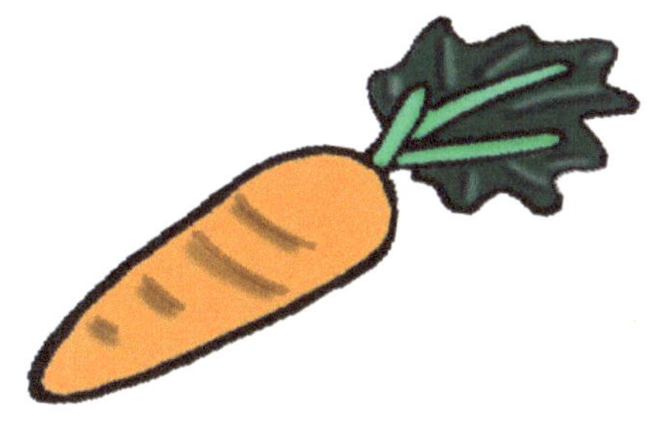

The poop train makes it all the way around to the other side and stops at the holding tank known as the *sigmoid colon.* The *sigmoid colon* announces really loud, even though we can't hear it... *"It's time to go to the bathroom!"*
The strong muscles of the *colon* squish and squish until your digested food waste we all call *poop* comes out.

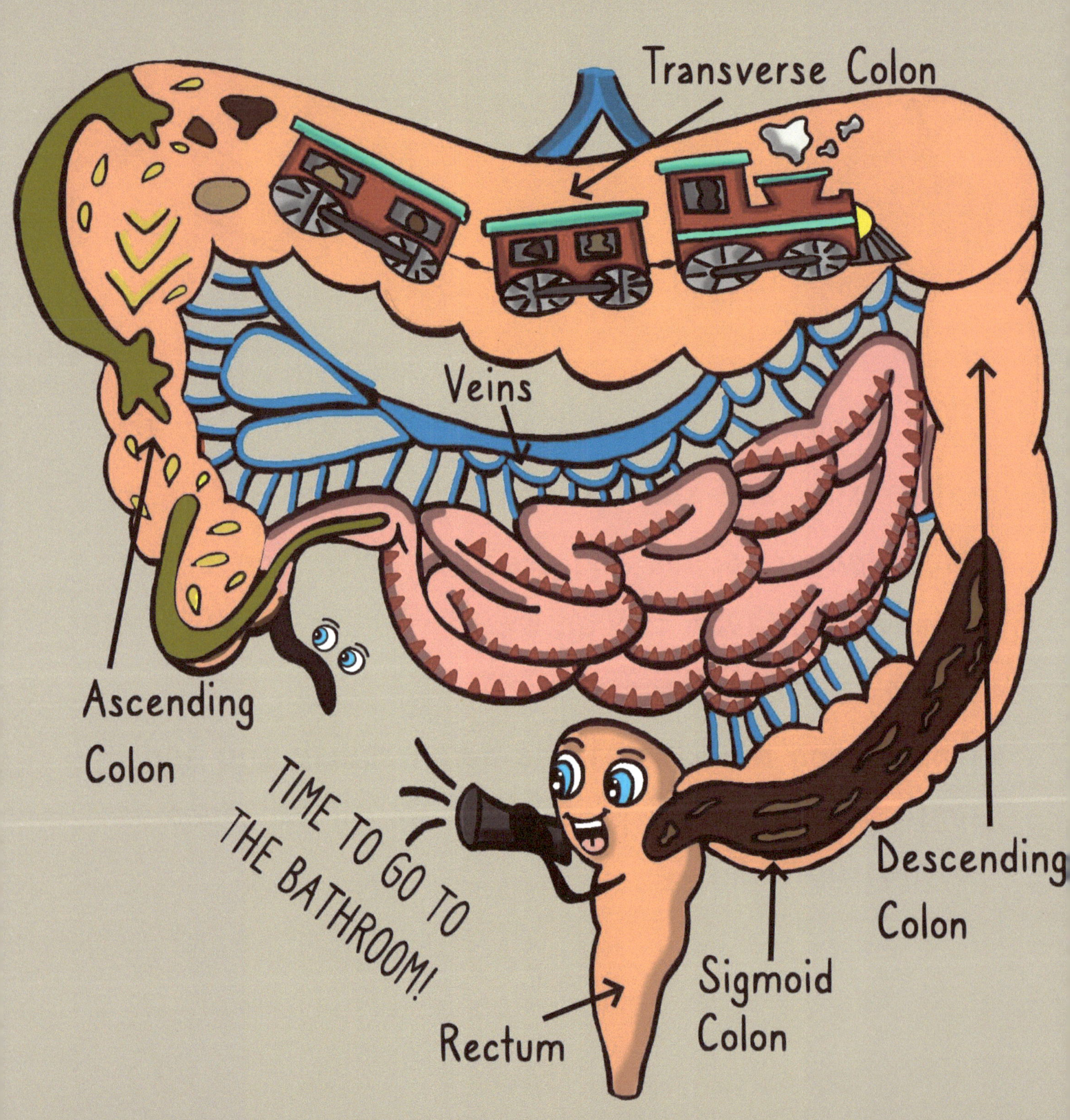

Transverse Colon
Veins
Ascending Colon
Descending Colon
Sigmoid Colon
Rectum
TIME TO GO TO THE BATHROOM!

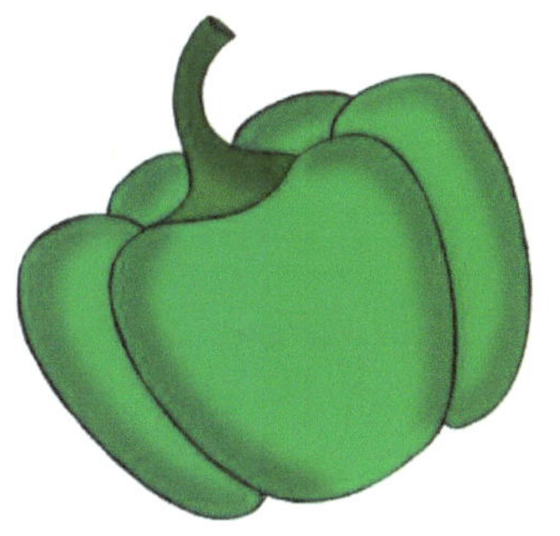

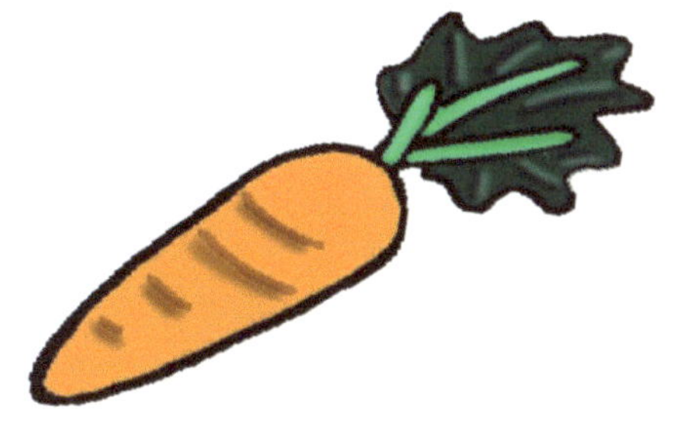

And that's where your food goes.
Now let's eat!"

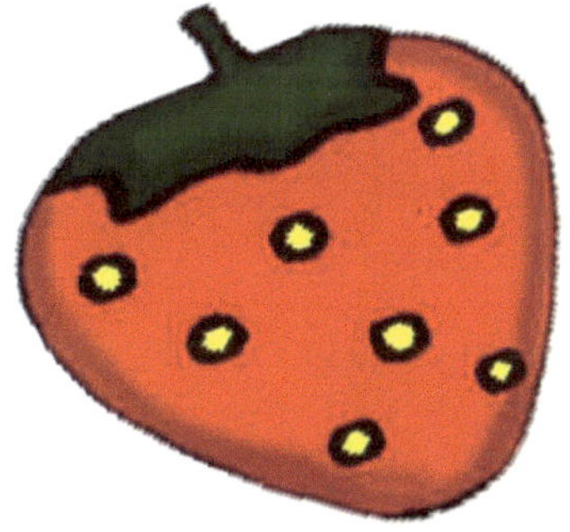

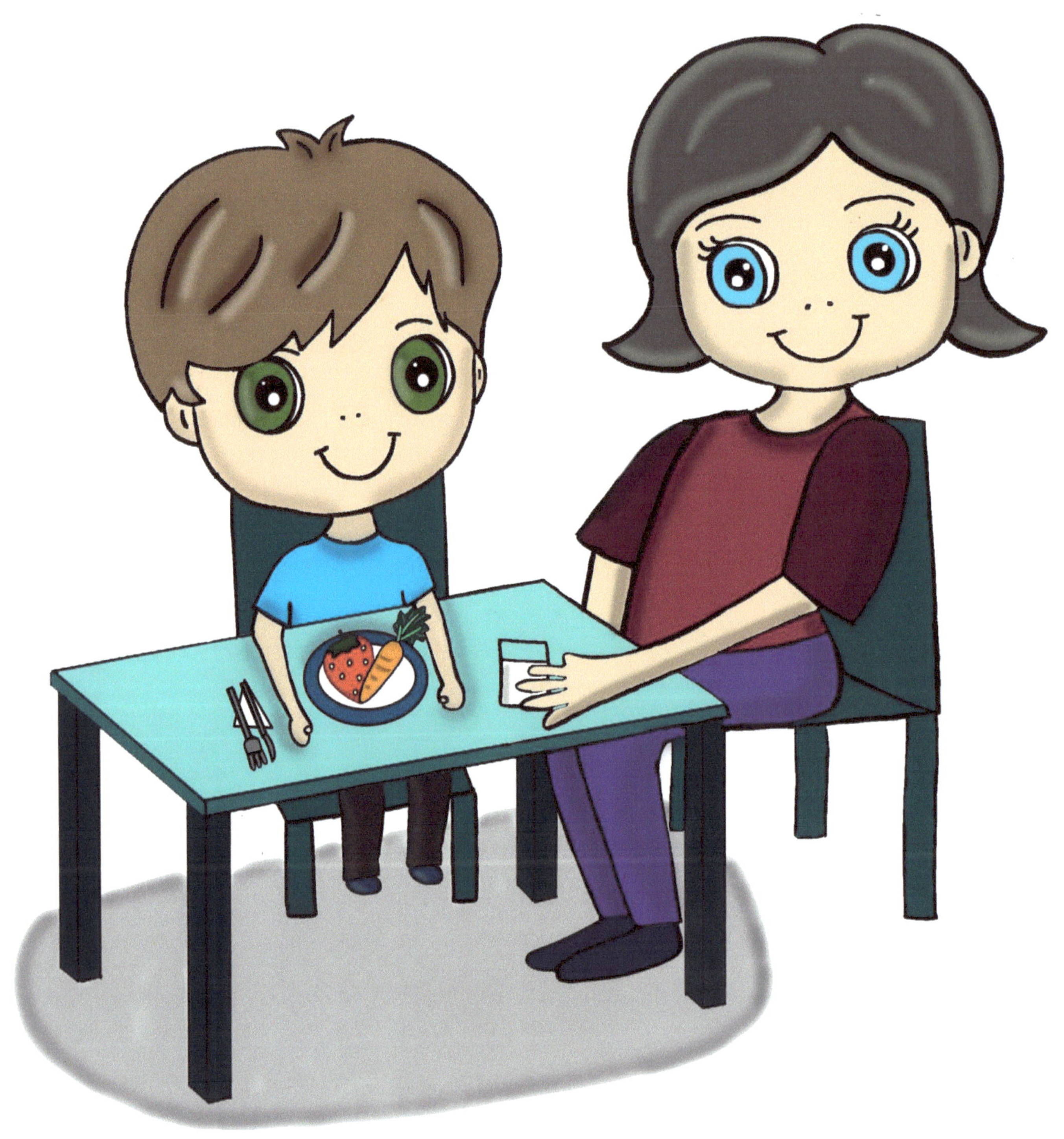